Senior Fitness:
Fit After 50

Learn How to Manage Your Fitness, Finances and Social Life in Retirement

RON KNESS

Table of Contents

Disclaimers

Introduction

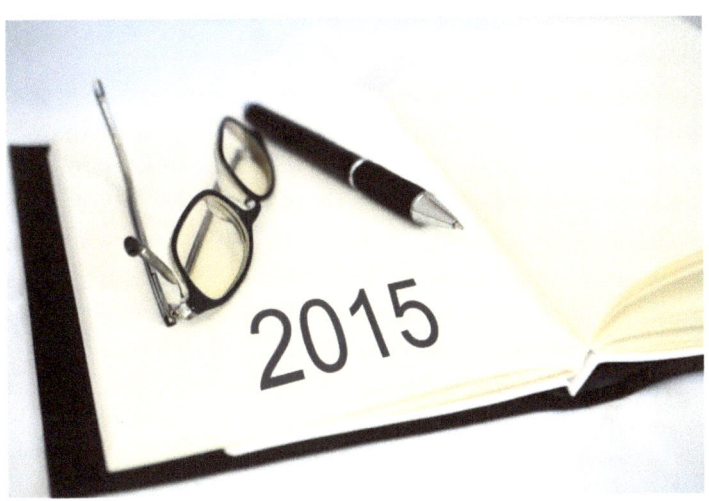

Shifting into an enjoyable retirement can come with a lot of challenges and obstacles – but it doesn't have to! When done properly, retirement can be an extremely enjoyable and pleasant experience. You just have to figure out how you can make the best of your retirement situation.

Some people have to have something to look forward to each day – a purpose for getting up, if you will. I'm one of those persons. For me, it was expanding my writing that I was doing on a part-time basis while still working. I always have at least a couple of writing projects in the works, so I know what I'm going to do each morning after getting up.

A large part of whether or not your retirement is enjoyable is how well you have planned for it financially.

Then of course the other part to this, is that you have managed to stay fit and healthy up to this point.

In this report we will look at ways that you can start to plan your retirement, early if you wish. This includes planning both financially, health wise and you will find tips about staying social.

Enjoy your read, on **_Senior Fitness – Fit After 50_**!

Ron Kness

http://healthylifestyle.ronkness.com/

knessr@gmail.com

Finances in Retirement – Assessing What You'll Need

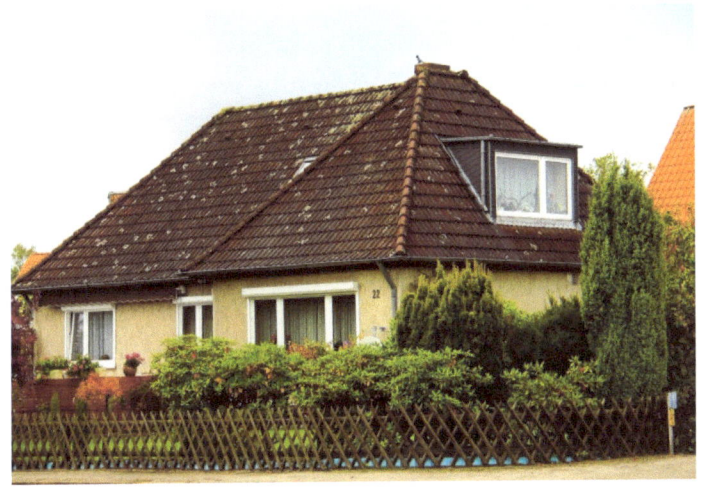

Whether you are just about to enter into retirement, or you are on the cusp and just looking to gain a heads up as to what you should expect, the first thing you will need to do is decide what sort of life you would like to have in retirement. There are a number of different ways to go about retirement, and no one way is right or wrong. However, how much money you have coming in each month in retirement will drive your decision in large part.

Which sort of retirement that is right for you? Well, that all depends on what you as a person will find fulfilling and enjoyable, as well as what your circumstances will permit. You could choose to remain in the same house you have lived in for years.

The house you have built a life in and have invested time and money; most likely it is paid for, so you wouldn't have a mortgage to worry about paying. Or you could sell your current house and decide to buy a smaller house, rent an apartment, or even move into a retirement community. Some sell everything and live full-time in an RV! While we had a senior condo in Minnesota after retiring, we did live in our 5th wheel 8 ½ months one year and 9 months the next. While on the road, we talked to many retirees whose only home was their RV and they loved the freedom of being able to move about whenever the travel bug bit them.

When assessing your finances to figure out exactly what sort of retirement is right, you will need to consider first how much money you have saved up. Do you have a 401K from your previous or current employer? Will you receive Social Security Benefits? Have you saved money back in your own savings account? Will you have other sources of income, such as a pension? These are all important questions to ask yourself.

After you have assessed how much money you have to retire on, you will then need to see if that fits your chosen retirement lifestyle. To do this you should make a list of monthly expenses. This list should include utilities, such as electric, gas, water, etc., as well as groceries, any monthly payments you have and some money for leisure activities.

By not commuting to work or having to wear office attire, buy lunch out, etc. those expenses should go down.

Then you will also need to estimate the number of years you will spend in retirement. With all of this added up and calculated, you will need to decide if your chosen retirement lifestyle is in your realm of possibilities. If it is not you have a few options. You can either choose a different, slightly more cost effective, life style – or you can up your retirement lifestyle to the one you dreamed of by doing a few different things.

If your current retirement savings aren't enough for you, there is always the option of investing. Many retired people choose this option regardless, because when entering into retirement your income becomes suddenly even more fixed than it was before.

Investing your money, if done properly, can give you the opportunity to stretch your retirement funds further. Generally the smart investment is one that will give you a guaranteed rate of return upon said investment. However you may need to invest more aggressively if your funds fall shockingly short. Generally it is a good idea to seek a one-time financial consultation either before you retire, or not long after you have entered into retirement.

Because time is your friend when investing, you should look to invest while still young and let it grow over time. While it may be too late for you to do this, it is a worthwhile tip to pass onto your kids and grandchildren; invest now and reap the benefits later.

Downsizing – Is It Right for You?

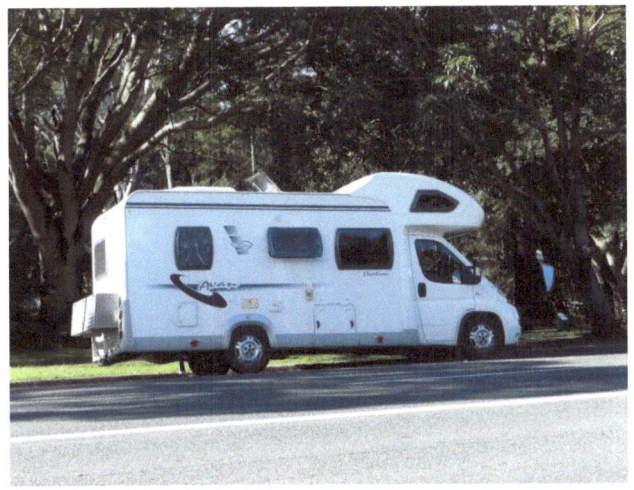

Downsizing is also another way to enhance your retirement lifestyle. Though the term downsizing does seem to carry with it a rather negative connotation it doesn't have to be a negative experience. When done properly, downsizing can be a worthwhile and fulfilling experience. It can also help you to achieve a more fruitful retirement lifestyle.

We downsized early – about 11 years before retiring. We sold our four-bedroom four-level house on a corner lot and with the equity we had in the house, we were able to buy a senior condo. With no mortgage to pay, a smaller place to maintain and no lawn to keep up, we were able to save a considerable amount of money over those last 11 years of working.

There are many ways and opportunities to downsize. The first being with your possessions. Getting rid of excess clutter and freeing up space in your home is not only a good way to relive some of the burden off of you, but also to make your home easier to navigate in the coming years and months.

When it comes to downsizing your possessions there are a few ways to go about it. First children and grandchildren love to inherit. Which means that when you are going through your possessions if there is anything that you would like to have out of the way but, can't bear to toss it in the trash or just give it to the Salvation Army, odds are that there is a child or grandchild who would love to have a family heirloom.

For those possessions that are just going to be in the way and have no real sentimental value to you there are options for getting rid of them as well. A yard sale is a great way to unload your clutter while also making a small bit of money to contribute towards your desired retirement lifestyle. Another option is to donate them to your local Goodwill or Salvation Army. This will take a burden off of you while also helping your community. And you may be able to take it off your taxes as a charitable donation, if you need the deduction.

Downsizing your home is also another potentially beneficial option. The term downsizing in reference to your home can mean something as small as getting rid of excess possessions, as mentioned above – or it could mean moving to a smaller more cost effective home. What this term will mean for you depends upon the various factors mentioned in the above text. As I said earlier, that is what we did only 11 years before we retired. It paid off handsomely!

If it does entail moving into a different home, either for a change of location, or for the benefits of a smaller abode, you will need to assess which option will be best for you. Many people choose to buy a smaller house in their retirement, or even to begin renting again. Both of these options have their advantages.

Moving into a smaller home will not only lower (or even wipe out entirely) your mortgage payment, but will also lower your utilities and the amount of time, effort, and money it will cost for upkeep and maintenance for your home and property.

Renting will give you the same advantages as a smaller house while also giving you added benefits of not having to pay property taxes, as well as not having to worry about maintenance and upkeep of the property, although in most cases you lose the flexibility of remodeling.

Retirement villages are also a great option for you to consider. Moving into a retirement village will have the same advantages as a smaller home and renting but will also offered added amenities (including social interaction) that may not otherwise be available to you.

Most retirement villages will offer shuttle buses to and from shops or events; this can save you money of fuel and car expenses. They will also, more often than not, offer community events, groups, and clubs that you are able to participate in, making it easy to stay involved, make new friends and socialize.

One of the most important things to remember when planning for retirement is to make sure you plan as far into the future as is possible. You need to consider how you will be able to get around your home in the coming years. Do you have stairs? Are your doorways wide enough to accommodate wheelchairs? Is it too cluttered to move about freely? All of these things could become obstacles that will require you to make adjustments or even move in the future.

Aging and Retirement – Smoothing Out the Emotional Roller Coaster

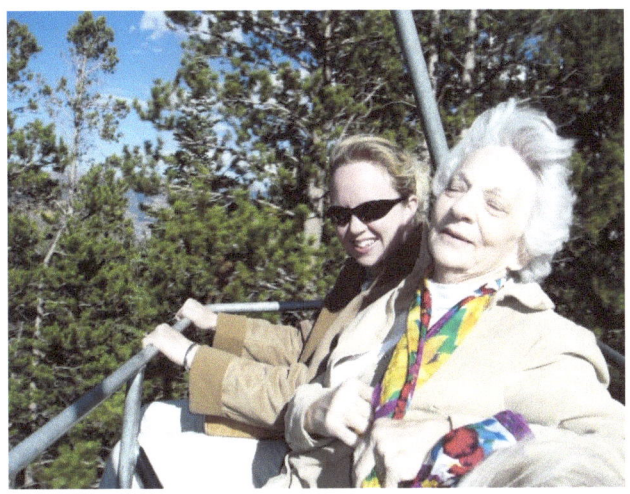

Many people fail to think of the emotional aspects of aging and retirement as well as the importance of staying social. Maintaining a healthy emotional level and social life will help you to get the most out of your retirement years.

There are many aspects of retirement that can affect your emotions. First and foremost is the loss of your sense of purpose. Without the requirement to get up and go to work every day, it is probable that you will no longer feel a sense of purpose. Or you may not feel as though you need to get up and get out of the house anymore.

There is also the risk of losing your sense of self. This is especially the case amongst many retired people today because we tend to define ourselves by our job – more so in men than women. You may believe that who you are is what you do. Losing this sense of self and purpose can lead to questions about your life in retirement as well as possible depression.

The benefits of staying social in retirement

Another problem is that you can lose your connection to your friends and the community. Especially if many of your friends are work-related friends whom you may not see as often now that you are not working with them every day. Losing all of these connections all at once can be disconcerting and even traumatic.

Staying social is a great way to maintain your emotional health in retirement. The benefits of maintaining your social connections throughout retirement – and especially in the beginning of your transition into retirement – can be immense. It could help you to adjust better and more quickly to the retirement lifestyle. Social engagement has also been shown to aid in your physical and mental health as well!

The social opportunities available to you are nearly endless, although depending on where you live and your physical condition you may have to rule out certain activities. However most towns will have a senior citizens center that will sponsor social events for the seniors in your town. These are a wonderful way to meet new people and perhaps even make a few friends. If you live in a retirement communities, social opportunities will be nearly at your fingertips 24/7!

Most retirement communities will hold potlucks, fun days, sponsored trips and even have groups available that meet on site. This means that in order to stay social, you won't have to travel outside of your community – which is a wonderful benefit if you have mobility problems; or you just don't enjoy traveling to do things.

If you don't live in a retirement community you can still find clubs that are of interest to you – however you will most likely have to look for them. They won't just be handed to you in a brochure. Still you have plenty of opportunities to be social.

Volunteering is beneficial to you and your community in many different ways. First, it allows you to maintain a social life, while also giving you a sense of purpose and fulfillment. It gives you the opportunity to engage socially with many different people and enrich both your life and theirs at the same time.

One of my friends that retired at the same time as I, immersed himself into several volunteering opportunities and stays as busy as he wants.

You have many options available when it comes to volunteering, you could help out at your local soup kitchen, tutor children after school, become a part of your neighborhood library's read to the youth program, or community betterment projects. It just depends on what interests you and what you would prefer to do. Habitat for Humanity is a great cause to be a part of.

Honestly, it doesn't matter how you choose to go about staying socially active, the important thing is that you do it. We, as humans, are social creatures by nature and maintaining that need is integral in the later years of your life when you lose some of your social connections due to retirement.

As Your Body Changes, So Should Your Diet

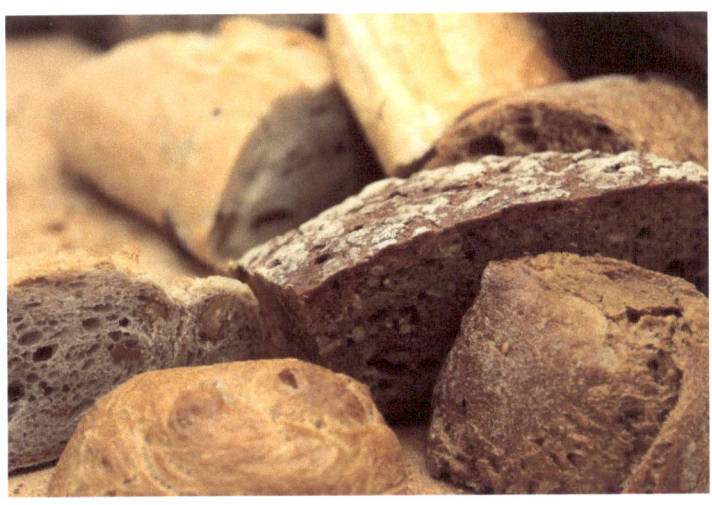

As your age changes, so should your body's nutrient needs. How you will absorb your nutrients can, and in most individuals do, change, along also with the ways in which you ingest them will change as well. Most retired individuals tend to eat less take out and more home cooked and healthy food. Which is good because you will need to start eating more nutrient dense foods and less processed and fast food loaded with saturated fat, salt and sugar.

Nutrient dense foods are simply foods that offer you the most bang for your buck. In other words they have a comparatively low calorie count, but high in nutrition.

These kinds of foods become increasingly important as you age because your body will require less calories, as you will not be working as much and your metabolism will most likely slow down, but you will need more nutrients to avoid a nutrient deficiency.

While taking vitamins can help you avoid such a deficiency, it is always better to get all of your essential vitamins, minerals, and nutrients though your diet, rather than from a daily pill. Your body is made to absorb nutrients from food. This means that it is easier on your body, and better for you if you can work with your body's natural digestive methods for nutrient absorption. You will get the most out of your diet that way.

Some examples of nutrient dense foods include, but are not limited to:

- Colorful and vibrant fruits and vegetables that are fresh, frozen, canned, dried, or even juiced!

- Lean meat, or meat with a lower fat content, including skinless poultry and fish; eggs, and beans are also great ways to get healthy protein with low calorie and fat content.

You will also generally need more calcium (especially if you are a women) than you did at previous points in life. Low fat, and even zero fat milk, yogurt, and cheese will all be wonderful ways to obtain your higher calcium needs while still managing to keep calorie and fat content low.

Fiber is also an important nutrient your body will require more of. Foods that are high in fiber but have a low calorie content in comparison are whole grains, such as certain breads and oatmeal, certain cereals, and even whole wheat pasta. Increasing your fiber and making sure you ingest it naturally will help your digestive system function more regularly and productively.

You will need to make sure you have a varied diet. The more variety you can include in meals and snacks, the better off you will be – especially when it comes to avoiding a nutrient deficiency. By eating a varied diet you will also be eating varied and complete nutrition, which is essential to maintaining your health in retirement.

Ease up on your junk food and 'extras' intake. This means you should avoid eating food items that contain excess calories and lack proper nutrition. This also goes for what you drink. It is recommended to drink as much water as possible and to limit your intake of other beverages such as soda in order to maintain health and avoid potential diet-related health problems in your future.

While there aren't many differences between women and men in retirement there are a few when it comes to how they adjust when entering retirement and their health requirements while in retirement that were worth mentioning.

Retirement – The Venus and Mars Factor in Women and Men

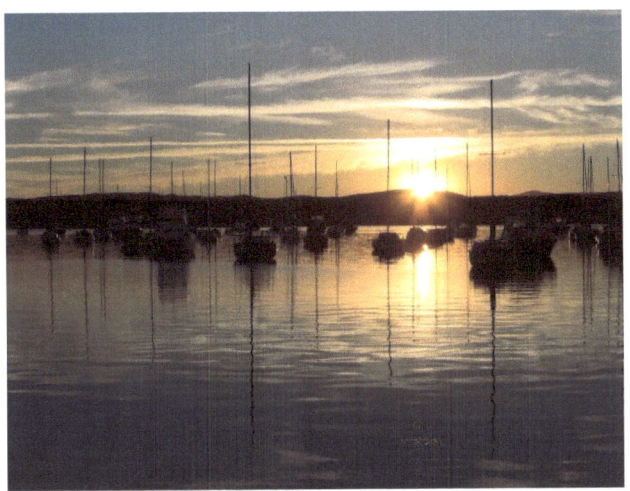

Women

For women retirement is in some ways easier than it is for men, while at the same time certain aspects of retirement are likely to be more challenging. For the most part, women have a generally easier time acclimating to the retirement lifestyle. This is due in part to the fact that they are usually more involved socially and have a wider social circle that extends beyond just their place of employment.

This allows women to have an easier time adjusting because they don't lose all of their social connections upon retirement. That, combined with their usual propensity to identify themselves by more than just the job, makes them far more adaptable to retirement.

This being said, women are still susceptible to questions about self and identity; they are just usually more adept and equipped to deal with them in a healthy way.

Women will also have certain differences in dietary needs – especially as they progress into their retirement years. Most women tend to lack enough iron and calcium in their diet. They will need make sure and pay special attention to these two requirements and eat foods fortified with iron and calcium.

Men

Men, like many women, will question their sense of self during retirement. The difference is that men do not typically deal with it as well as women do. Some of them take much longer to adjust to this new lifestyle. Questions such as, who am I?, and what is my purpose? tend to plague men longer than women.

The reason it will generally take men longer to adjust is because society today has typically defined men by what they do. So, in turn, men tend to define themselves in the same way – by their work. Once the work is gone, so can their self-identity. Also, men do not tend to have social circles with as wide of berths as women do.

Many times a man's social circle will not extend beyond his work place. The loss of his job and his social circle at the same time can be startling.

The stress associated with this can cause severe emotional unbalance in men. They also usually have trouble adjusting to being home more, they may feel as though they have no purpose, nothing to drive them. They may not know where they fit in their life anymore.

One of the easiest and best ways to rectify this is to become active in a social activity of some sort – before retiring if you can, so that you are established upon retiring. Find a club or hobby that you will enjoy, or used to enjoy, and begin doing it again. Perhaps finding old hobbies that you enjoyed once and just didn't have the time for while you worked. You will have enough time now that you no longer have to worry about time constraints due to your being employed. I was able to take up **fly rod building** (http://www.amazon.com/Making-Your-First-Fly-Rod-ebook/dp/B00DQGMO7W) after I retired and start **tying my own fishing flies** (http://www.amazon.com/Beginners-Guide-Fly-Tying-ebook/dp/B00DRES2LA) once again – something I had done as a teenager and enjoyed.

Men also tend to worry more about finances in retirement given that they are no longer bringing in as much money each month and their income is suddenly more fixed than it was before retirement; this too can lead to increased stress. They worry that they won't have enough money, or that if a situation arises, they may not have the money necessary to deal with it.

However, this fear is not singular as it pertains to women as well; it is just more prevalent in retired men than in their female counterparts. They also may feel diminished because they are no longer providing for their household by going to work every day.

Planning for the future and perhaps even seeking financial advice (highly recommended) in regards to your retirement, whether you are already in retirement or just about to enter into this glorious chapter in your life, could go a long way towards abating those fears as it offers everyone involved reassurance and peace of mind.

Maintaining Your Physical and Social Activity in Retirement

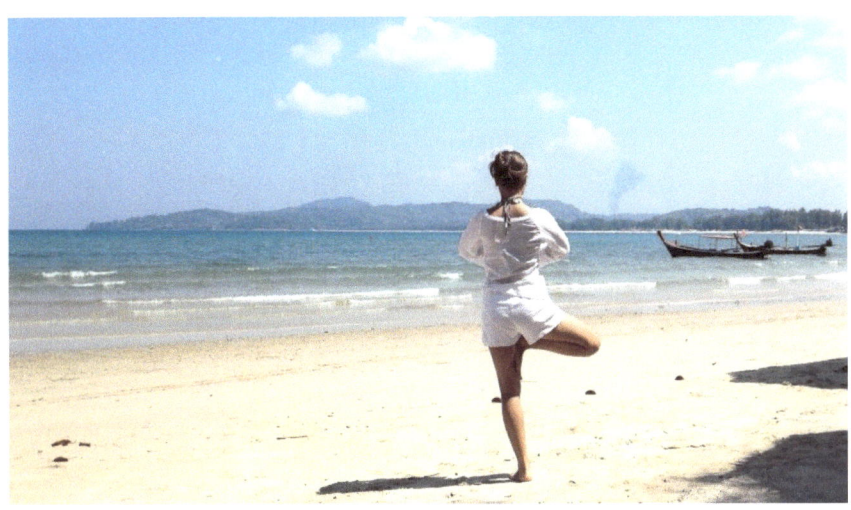

Regular exercise increasingly becomes extremely important as we age. It doesn't matter if you have never exercised before in your life, the fact of the matter is, the older you get the more important and beneficial it is to exercise. Partaking in regular exercise will help you stay healthy; not only physically, but also emotionally and mentally as well.

For most adults in retirement exercise is physically beneficial because it can help relieve joint pain and stiffness, as well as keep your body moving, and working. Not only will exercise keep or even increase joint flexibility, it can also preserve the muscle you have and diminish muscle mass loss in the future – something that happens at the rate of 10% per decade after age 50 if left unchecked.

This will allow you to be as independent as possible (for as long as possible) when it comes to getting around your house and anywhere else you may wish to go.

It also helps with mental and emotional health by producing happy hormones. When you exercise regularly your body produces the hormone endorphin, along with others, that promote positive emotions and mental health. Regular physical activity, combined with activities that require you to think a little bit have been proven to improve and prolong mental competency in retired adults.

Which type of exercise is right for you? Well that depends on your level of physical fitness as well as what your body will allow you to do. If you did work out before retirement and you can no longer do your chosen activity, you should replace it with a similar activity that is within your body's means. It is always a good idea to consult your physician before beginning any type of exercise regimen to ensure that your body can handle the stress of the exercise you are about to undertake.

Hiking and **walking** (http://www.amazon.com/Design-Your-Ultimate-Fitness-Program-ebook/dp/B00S4ALBMO) are both great exercises that many retired adults are able to do and even enjoy! They are great for your overall health, mental, emotional, and physical.

Hiking and **walking**
(http://www.amazon.com/Walking-Down-Road-Fitness-Healthy-ebook/dp/B00PD8B6ES) are low impact aerobic exercises that can promote cardiovascular and muscle health.

These are the perfect activities to be done with your spouse or friend that will get you up and moving and also get you outside and into nature. You can walk around your neighborhood, or the local park. You could hike the trails at said park, or depending on the area in which you live, you may even have access to other hiking trails.

Aside from the physical benefits of walking the emotional and psychological benefits are exponential. Being outside and in nature and just getting away for a small while, either on your own or with another person, promotes a healthy emotional and psychological well-being. It will also help you to have a reason to leave the house and get up and around.

Water aerobics is also another extremely good exercise for many various reasons. The first being that it far easier on your body than traditional aerobics and weight training exercises. Also, the beauty of water aerobics is that even though it is more low impact than weight training the resistance of the water acts like weights, allowing you to work out more efficiently with less physical stress.

It is also a great way for you to stay social, as water aerobics are generally conducted in a class or group setting. This means that you can interact with other adults, as well as bring your friends to workout with you. Although my wife and I have our own pool and play an hour of volleyball most days. With only two people, it is a workout!

If your body is able enough to handle it, off road biking can be another activity you may want to look into. It is cardiovascular and strength training all at once, meaning you can kill two birds with one stone while also having fun and possibly exploring new destinations.

Many places will offer biking trails for off road biking either in their park – or perhaps if you are lucky enough, a wooded area inside or around town. This, just as with hiking, gets you outside with purpose and can be done on your own or with a spouse, friend, and even a group of friends.

Swimming is a low impact full body workout that will also work your cardiovascular system at the same time as it is strengthening your muscle groups. Swimming is a total physical workout that will get your heart rate up and your muscles moving.

However if you have not swam in a while, or you are quick to tire while swimming it is a good idea to make sure you have another person with you at all times for safety. You need to take care to pay special attention to your body when swimming and don't overtire yourself because this increases your chance of water-related risks.

Not all of the activities you partake in during your retirement need to be purely exercise oriented, it is good practice to engage in non-physical social activities as well as activities that are relaxing and engaging to your mind.

Bird watching is one such example. While typically a sedentary activity, it is still a beneficial activity that you may find enjoyable. It can be a social activity as well, if you perhaps find other bird watching enthusiasts in your area you can do it with – or even your area may have a local bird watching club that meets regularly to share photos or discuss what sort of birds they have seen recently.

This is an example of a mental and socially stimulating activity that will rely little on your mobility. So long as you are able to sit by a window, or on a bench in a park you should have no problem bird watching.

Another great activity that you may find enjoyable is gardening. **Gardening** (http://www.amazon.com/Gardening-Your-Way-Fitness-Healthful-ebook/dp/B00WKU66U6) can have numerous and nearly endless benefits for you and your household. If you choose to gardening can become an integral part of your retirement lifestyle. It can help you with everything from downsizing, health, and activity.

However this all depends on what you choose to plant. If you have a vegetable and herb garden, then you could cut your grocery bill down, while also ensuring that the food you are eating is free of GMO's, pesticides, and other chemicals. Growing your own vegetables allow you to have a greater amount of control over your diet – at least for certain times of the year.

Perhaps you would rather just have a garden that is aesthetically pleasing, instead of nutritional. This is OK as well, there are no rules saying which sort of gardening you should be doing in retirement, if you so choose to. Flower gardens can create a lovely place to sit and relax during the day, as well as possibly attracting birds for watching.

Gardening is also an activity that you can do at your own pace and leisure. Your garden can be as large, or as small, or as intricate, or simple as you desire. It all depends on what you want, and what you and your body are capable of handling.

While gardening can be a perfectly pleasing solitary activity, it can easily be turned into a social activity as well. There are many ways to go about becoming social in gardening, you could volunteer at a community garden, or you could start/join a gardening club nearby.

Volunteering at your local community garden will benefit both you and your community immensely. First, it allows you to feel a sense of connection with your community as a whole, and can also help you to feel valued as an individual – both of which are extremely important parts of a successful retirement.

Perhaps, if you're local community does not have a community garden, you could find a few people in your neighborhood or the surrounding neighborhoods to form a gardening club. It's another way to make gardening into a social activity while also possibly learning new things about it as well as the people in your club.

The activities we have mentioned are by no means the only activities available to you as a retired individual; there are and endless amount of physical and social opportunities for you to partake in. It is all about getting out there and finding what you are capable of and what you are interested in and turning those into something you can actively participate in for the coming years.

In the End ...

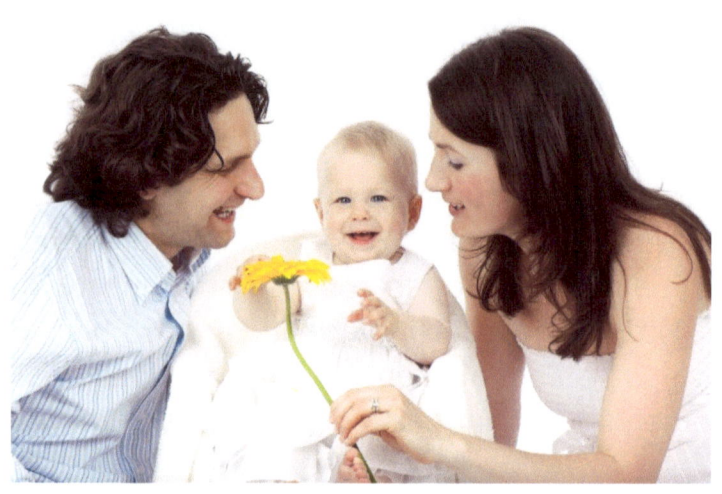

Retirement can seem to be a daunting and stressful time in your life; it can seem like one of those things that you have no clue how to go about and you may feel like you have nowhere to turn. However, it is important to remember the success tips we have outlined here, doing this will help to ensure you have an enjoyable retirement.

Remember that planning ahead will be one of the best things you can do, both for yourself, and your family. It will help everyone involved to feel reassured and hopeful in this period of great transition in your life, and the lives of those around you.

Aside from planning financially for your desired future, you should remember to eat healthy and stay active and social. The benefits of doing so will be nearly immeasurable as your life progresses. Staying positive and maintaining your social connections helps you to adjust to retirement smoother, and more quickly, than just trying to 'wing it' per say.

Enjoy yourself! This is a great time in your life.

Ron Kness

http://healthylifestyle.ronkness.com/

knessr@gmail.com

If you are interested in reading further about staying fit in your senior years, get my book *Senior Fitness – A Guide to Staying Young Beyond Your Years.*
(http://www.amazon.com/Senior-Fitness-Guide-Staying-Beyond-ebook/dp/B00Q04LVL2)

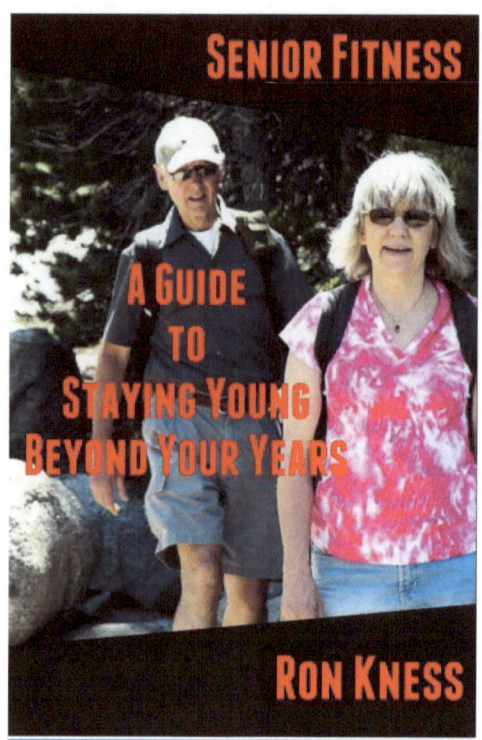

Other Books You May Be Interested In Purchasing

Many seniors are plagued with arthritis. In my book ***Arthritis – Live With Less Pain and Inflammation*** (*http://www.amazon.com/Arthritis-Live-Inflammation-Techniques-Lessen-ebook/dp/B00WAOH4JE*), I discuss tips and techniques that you can use to lessen the pain and swelling.

You learn things like:
• Simple and effective information that will help you manage the pain and inflammation that comes along with arthritis, so that you can live an active, full life without debilitating pain.
• The different types of arthritis, their symptoms and how to alleviate their painful side effects.
• The pros and cons of over-the-counter arthritis medications, plus simple tips that will help you know how to choose the right supplements.
• Free, yet effective ways to get relief from arthritis pain and inflammation, so you don't have to suffer anymore. The effects arthritis can have significant impact on your physical and mental well-being, but this book shows you how to overcome its painful symptoms and live life relatively pain free.

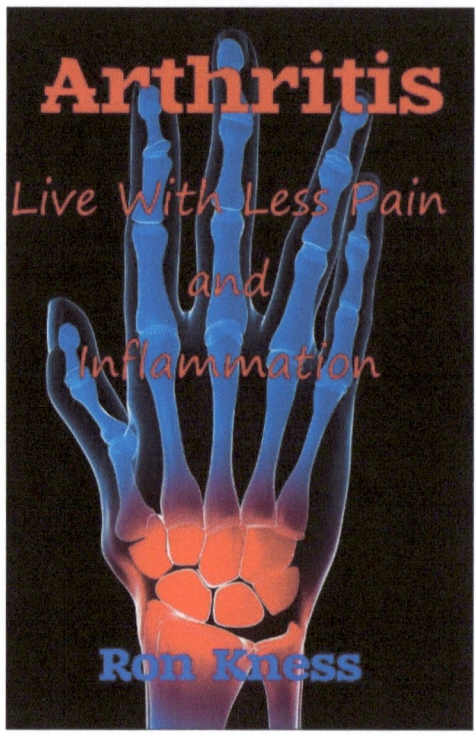

Gardening is a great activity many seniors like to do. Do you know it is also a great way to get exercise and get fit? It's true!

Isn't it time to get outdoors? The gym is a great place to stay fit during the colder seasons, but once the temperature turns warmer you want to spend more time outside. Plus, you'll have the benefit of fresh wholesome produce to enjoy by growing vegetables in your backyard garden.

Does this sound like your situation?
• You sit for hours at a desk at work.
• The hum of the overhead lights is a constant reminder you never go outdoors.
• Often you skip workouts because you want to spend the time with your family.
• Everyone in the family is overweight.
• You worry about declining health and are on edge and anxious.
• You know exercise would help, but you just don't have the energy or motivation.

Does it seem as if your destiny to live constantly indoors breathing recycled air under artificial lights?

Why not combine fitness and gardening to accomplish your healthy lifestyle goals?

Working in the garden provides a well-rounded workout. Think about all you accomplish with a workout in the garden:
• Gardening tasks improve your endurance, flexibility and strength.
• The food you grow is fresh providing wholesome nutrition for the family.
• Your family learns the process of planting, nurturing and harvesting the food they eat.
• A 30 minute garden workout burns more calories than 30 minutes running.
• Everyone enjoys the satisfaction of participating in a project from start to finish.

People are turning to hobby gardening as a way to burn off stress while getting back in touch with the basics of living. They also find that gardening tasks like raking, hoeing and digging is very slimming! But there are benefits beyond burning calories and firming muscles. Outdoor activity reduces anxiety, too. Studies have shown a link between ADHD and insufficient outdoors time. Senior living homes include an outdoor sanctuary where residents benefit from simple gardening activities to keep mind and body engaged.

Introducing "*Gardening Your Way to Fitness - The Fun Way to Get Fit and Provide Beauty and Healthful Bounty for Your Family*" (http://www.amazon.com/Gardening-Your-Way-Fitness-Healthful-ebook/dp/B00WKU66U6).

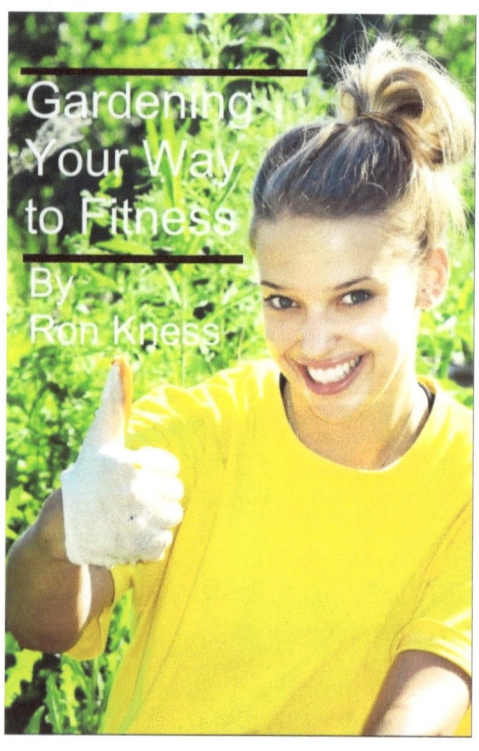

About the Author

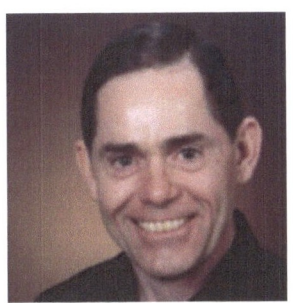

I grew up in Central Minnesota, where my parents own and operated a fishing resort. Once out of high school I tried a couple of semesters of college, only to quit halfway through the Spring term; I decided at that time that college wasn't for me.

Then I decided to follow my father's previous occupation as an auto mechanic. I graduated from a two-year of vocational training course and worked as a mechanic. While in vocational training, I decided to join the National Guard where I eventually ended up working full-time for 32 years.

So how does all of this relate to writing? In one of my leadership schools, the instructor, who was an English teacher at a juvenile detention center, presented writing to me in a whole new way - a way that started to develop my interest in working with words.

Fast forward about 40 years and I now have over 20 books listed on Amazon for Kindle. All of my books with the exception of one children's book (One, Two, Three, Four . . . Counting is Fun at the Grocery Store) are non-fiction in various fields, such as:

*Health and Fitness:

- What You Eat Can Hurt You

- Eat Healthy to Lose Weight

- The Extreme Weight Loss Plan

- Get Ripped Abs

- Walking Down the Road to Fitness

- Design Your Ultimate Fitness Program - Walking

- A Healthier You in the Coming Year

- Senior Fitness – A Guide to Staying Young Beyond Your Years

- Managing Type 2 Diabetes Using Alternative And Natural Therapies

SENIOR FITNESS – FIT AFTER 50

RON KNESS

- The No Nonsense Guide to Digital Photography

- The Beginner's Guide to Digital Photography

- Digital Photography – A Quick Guide to Using Adobe Photoshop Elements

- Improve Your Blog Posts With Photos

- Digital Photography Anthology

* Travel:
- Travel Advisor

- Travel Trips and Tips

*Outdoors and Recreation:

- Making Your First Fly Rod

- The Beginner's Guide to Fly Tying

- Hooked on Fly Fishing

- The Secrets to Fly Fishing for Trout

- Tent Camping – The Ultimate in Family Fun

- Maintaining a Salt Water Pool

* Misc.:

- Making Wine from Kits

- Create Your Home Inventory

- The 9 Secrets to Using Your GI Bill Benefits

- The Life and Times of the Honey Bee

- The Military Spouses Financial Guide to Funding Education

- The Home-Based Entrepreneur's Guide to Blogging

- Survival Basics – Are You Prepared to Survive?

Besides my own writing, I also ghostwrite ebooks, reports, articles, blogs and do Kindle conversions for my clients.

Oh . . . did I mention that I went back to college in 1987 and graduated 7 years later?

Today my wife and I live in Gold Canyon, AZ, where you'll find me happily sitting in my office typing away on my laptop as I work on my next book or ghostwriting project . . . that is if we are not traveling on a cruise ship - our new-found mode of travel.

If you like my books, please leave a review of them on Amazon at the book links where purchased.